GW01316168

# Blood Circulation Problems

## How to Improve Blood Circulation for a Healthier Body

by Maureen Knapp

# Table of Contents

# Introduction

Blood circulation problems can cause major issues for the different human body systems. This is because blood circulation acts as the network that supplies oxygen, hemoglobin, and other essential nutrients to all the cells and tissues in the body. You can easily understand this if you think about it as a water system supplying water to the various parts of your city. If problems occur in this system, then individuals can die because of lack of water.

When the blood circulation system in your body is dysfunctional, this can result in the death of your cells and eventually, in the deterioration of your overall health. Therefore, it's imperative that you keep this system unimpaired and flowing smoothly in order to maintain your health and well-being.

As the cliché goes, prevention is better than cure. It's crucial that you know how to prevent blood circulation problems from happening. This is to ensure that your systems can work properly and reliably. In cases where blood circulation problems exist already, they must be addressed promptly to avoid further damage to your cells.

This book will present numerous methods by which you can improve your blood circulation so that future problems can be prevented. It will also help you in resolving blood circulation issues through various home management techniques and other effective methods. (And as with any potentially serious medical condition, a visit to your physician is always recommended.) Don't wait for things to get worse; get the information you need now to make improvements today.

© Copyright 2015 by Miafn LLC - All rights reserved.

This document is geared towards providing reliable information in regards to the topic and issue covered. The publication is sold with the idea that the publisher is not required to render accounting, officially permitted, or otherwise, qualified services. If advice is necessary, legal or professional, a practiced individual in the profession should be ordered.

- From a Declaration of Principles which was accepted and approved equally by a Committee of the American Bar Association and a Committee of Publishers and Associations.

In no way is it legal to reproduce, duplicate, or transmit any part of this document in either electronic means or in printed format. Recording of this publication is strictly prohibited and any storage of this document is not allowed unless with written permission from the publisher. All rights reserved.

The information provided herein is stated to be truthful and consistent, in that any liability, in terms of inattention or otherwise, by any usage or abuse of any policies, processes, or directions contained within is solely and completely the responsibility of the recipient reader. Under no circumstances will any legal responsibility or blame be held against the publisher for any reparation, damages, or monetary loss due to the information herein, either directly or indirectly.

Respective authors own all copyrights not held by the publisher.

The information herein is offered for informational purposes solely, and is universal as so. The presentation of the information is without contract or any type of guarantee assurance.

The trademarks that are used are without any consent, and the publication of the trademark is without permission or backing by the trademark owner. All trademarks and brands within this book are for clarifying purposes only and are the owned by the owners themselves, not affiliated with this document.

# Chapter 1: The Importance of Proper Blood Circulation

For you to be able to prevent blood circulation problems, it helps if you know the basic facts. Blood circulation is one of the functions of the circulatory system (comprising 3 individual systems): the cardiovascular (heart), the respiratory (lungs) and the systemic (blood vessels). Hence, if the circulatory system is dysfunctional, blood circulation problems will also arise. Here are the essential functions of blood circulation of which you should be aware.

## Importance of proper blood circulation

### Provides sufficient hemoglobin

The circulation of blood provides hemoglobin packed inside the Red Blood Cells (RBCs) to all cells and tissues in the body. Insufficient hemoglobin will cause several diseases that include anemia. Anemia, if left untreated, can lead to death.

### Provides essential nutrients

Through blood circulation, essential nutrients needed by your body's cells are brought to all parts of your body. Without proper nourishment, these cells will not be able to perform effectively. You can think of your body cells as construction workers inside your body. If they are hungry, they can't build your body well.

## Brings water to cells

It's also through the blood that water is brought to the cells for proper hydration. Cells need to be hydrated sufficiently so they can survive and function reliably.

## Transports gases

Oxygen and carbon dioxide are transported through blood circulation. These gases are converted into soluble forms and brought to where they are needed. Oxygen is delivered to the cells where it is required for respiration to take place, for cells to convert food into energy so they can survive.

Oxygen is transported in the form of oxyhemoglobin, while carbon dioxide goes through several conversions depending on the needs of your systems. If your body is acidic and needs more alkalinity, carbon dioxide is converted to the alkaline substance, bicarbonate. When the body is alkaline and needs more acidity, carbon dioxide combines with water to form carbonic acid. These processes are reversible based on the pH (acidity and alkalinity) of your blood.

The pH is determined by the amount of acid/alkali (or base) in a solution. For your body to maintain homeostasis it must retain a pH balance between 7.35 and 7.45. Any acid-base imbalance that is left untreated can cause coma, organ failure and then death.

**Transports waste products**

It's also through the blood circulation that waste products of metabolism are transported to be excreted from the body. Waste products are those that are not needed by the body such as urea, urobilin, urobilinogen, creatinine and excess water, electrolytes, sugar and bilirubin. If these toxic substances are not properly eliminated, they can cause toxicity and death.

**Transports regulatory molecules**

Regulatory molecules are hormones and enzymes which are in charge of regulating the state of balance of substances in your body (homeostasis). The hormones are "chemical messengers" that send messages to the brain so that certain biochemical reactions can be initiated, while enzymes are "accelerators" that hasten chemical reactions. When your enzymes and hormones are not transported by the blood circulation to the body part that is in dire need of it, this can lead to serious health problems.

### Regulates pH and osmosis

This is related to the transport of gases because carbon dioxide helps maintain the blood pH. The movement of water inside the body is likewise related to your blood circulation. Blood brings water to areas where it's needed.

### Transports processed molecules

Molecules, such as vitamin D, are transported through the blood from one organ to another in their precursor forms until, as in the example of vitamin D, it becomes active vitamin D. Important substances, such as amino acids and fatty acids, are also transported through the blood.

These are the major functions of blood circulation. If you notice, these are key functions that must be accomplished because they are crucial in keeping you alive.

# Chapter 2: Causes of Blood Circulation Problems

Because blood is the major transport system in your body, almost all diseases can affect your blood circulation. To aid you in coping with these problems, here are causes of blood circulation problems.

## Polycythemia vera

This is a condition in which there are more Red Blood Cells than normal. This makes the blood more "viscous". This increased viscosity of blood will make it harder for it to flow smoothly to the various parts of the body. Blood circulation becomes slow, affecting the speed of response to body emergencies.

## Venous thrombosis

This is the presence of thrombus or blood clots inside blood vessels that cause problems in blood circulation. The thrombi prevent blood from flowing to the affected body part. The blockage of your blood vessels causes the cells in that part of your body to die. This is a dangerous situation that requires prompt treatment.

## Thrombophlebitis

This is characterized by the inflammation of veins or arteries, impeding blood flow. This needs immediate medical treatment so consult your doctor right away.

## Thrombocytopenia

This is a condition characterized by the reduced number of platelets. When the number of platelets is greatly decreased, the blood thins and hemorrhaging may occur.

## Atherosclerosis

This is the formation of cholesterol plaques on the walls of your blood vessels. This accumulation of cholesterol will thicken the area. This will then reduce the circumference of the veins and arteries, thereby making it difficult for the blood to pass through. Consequently, the heart has to increase the pressure in pumping blood so that it can force the blood to pass through the smaller openings. This will abnormally increase your blood pressure.

Hypertension or elevated blood pressure can cause a cholesterol plaque to suddenly rupture and the sudden blood clot that ensues increases your risk of cardiac illnesses, such as myocardial infarction (MI) or heart attack, and cerebrovascular accidents (CVA) or stroke. Unmanaged hypertension can also damage your kidneys, brain, and the other vital organs in your body. This could prove fatal.

## Arteriosclerosis

This is the smaller version of atherosclerosis because the lipid affected areas are your small arteries. But the effect is just as severe as atherosclerosis. You should also visit your doctor in this case.

## Vertebrobasilar circulatory disorder

This is a disorder caused by poor blood circulation in the back of the neck. Since the brain is significantly affected by the lack of oxygen, this can cause a myriad of symptoms.

## Stress

Stress can lead to poor blood circulation because stress can trigger hormones that disrupt the existing balance (homeostasis) of your body. The catecholamine hormones (epinephrine and norepinephrine) are increased in secretion to respond to your stress mode. These are your emergency hormones that are responsible for your "flight" or "fight" response during stressful situations. They usually constrict your arteries and increase your blood pressure. They also increase your other vital signs namely; Respiration Rate (RR), Pulse Rate (PR), and Heart Rate (HR). These affect the circulation of your blood.

The hormone glucocorticoid is also increased during stress. The increased secretion of this hormone can cause a myriad of health problems including circulation problems. The hormone increases sugar in your bloodstream that can cause increased viscosity.

## Raynaud's disease

This is caused by the narrowing of the blood vessels in the extremities (legs, arms), lips, ears and nipples during cold weather or during extremely stressful situations.

## Peripheral arterial disease (PAD)

This is similar to Raynaud's, but the narrowing of the blood vessels is caused by hardening of the vessels because of fat deposits.

## Tight fitting clothes

This is a physiological cause of poor circulation. This can simply be remedied by loosening your clothing. Imagine pressing a water hose—that's exactly what you're doing with your blood vessels when you wear tight-fitting clothes.

## Insufficient exercise

When you don't get enough exercise, you don't burn the fats in your body. These fats tend to accumulate on the walls of your veins and arteries resulting to atherosclerosis (mentioned above). This condition will affect your blood circulation by clogging your blood vessels. Exercising increases the flow of blood that flushes out those fat particles from your blood vessels.

These are the major causes of blood circulation problems. Problems in blood circulation are the effects of these diseases. You must remember this so that you can easily understand the coping mechanism and prevention techniques presented in the next chapters.

# Chapter 3: Symptoms Related to Circulation Problems

Become familiar with the symptoms of blood circulation problems, so you can deal with them appropriately. Two of the most common problems are poor circulation and blocked blood vessels. Again, these conditions can lead to organ failure and then death.

## Symptoms of blood circulation problems

### Heaviness and pain in the affected area

The extremities (legs and arms) often suffer from poor or blocked circulation, in which case you will experience pain and heaviness in these extremities. You may also have difficulty moving them.

### Feeling numb or cold

Sometimes, you won't feel pain and heaviness, but you will be numb with cold instead. When numbness or coldness sets in, it denotes that the blood circulation may have been completely obstructed. If the body part involved is turning a black or bluish color, then this is a life-threatening situation—that limb may have to be amputated before it affects the rest of the body. Swift action is needed to prevent the loss of body parts.

Poor circulation can be caused by fat deposits or plaques in the blood vessels of these extremities. This is called Peripheral Vascular Disease (PVD). If you are a high-risk individual, be constantly on the lookout for these symptoms.

## Change of color of extremity to pale, blue or black

In extreme cases, the affected area may turn blue and cells can die unless treatment measures are initiated. Therefore, you have to observe for any paleness, hematoma (bluish color of extremity) or black color of any part of your body, and report this to your doctor immediately.

## Tingling of extremities

In some individuals, poor circulation is manifest in the tingling of the extremities. This can feel like a thousand tiny needles pricking your skin.

These are the physical symptoms of blood circulation problems. Keep in mind that when illnesses are causing the problems, you have to expect that the symptoms of that specific illness will also become evident. For example, when the cause of poor circulation is polycythemia vera (a bone marrow disorder responsible for heightened production of red blood cells), you can also expect to observe the symptoms of polycythemia vera.

## Polycythemia vera symptoms

- Increased Erythrocyte Sedimentation Rate (ESR)—normal is 0–22 mm/hr. for men, and 0–29 mm/hr. for women)—a lab test is done to determine if your Red Blood Cells (RBCs) are normal.
- Headache
- Dizziness
- Dyspnea when lying down—difficulty in breathing
- Itchiness—usually after a shower
- Fatigue
- Joint inflammations
- Skin rashes

## Symptoms of atherosclerosis and arteriosclerosis

- Elevated blood cholesterol levels, above 200 mg/dL (cholesterol levels are measured in milligrams (mg) of cholesterol per deciliter (dL) of blood)

- Hypertension

## Thrombocytopenia symptoms

- Propensity for bleeding (internal and external)
- Various hematoma on skin
- Low platelet count (normal count is 150,000 to 400,000/cumm (per cubic millimeter)
- Prolonged bleeding time (BT) and clotting time (CT)

**For venous thrombosis and thrombophlebitis,** the symptoms may not be apparent physically, except for the skin changing color to blue or black.

## The symptoms of peripheral arterial disease (PAD)

- Cold extremities
- Tingling
- Numbness
- Pain

## Symptoms of vertebrobasilar circulatory disorder

This is one of the complications of stroke and has symptoms such as:

- Blurred vision
- Difficulty in walking
- Headache
- Nausea and vomiting
- Urinary and bowel control can become problematic
- Inability to maintain balance
- Slurred speech
- Difficulty in swallowing

## Symptoms of stress

For problems in blood circulation caused by stress, you may experience the following symptoms:

- Insomnia
- Hyperventilation
- Indigestion
- Headaches
- Stomachaches
- Weakness
- Dizzy spells
- Nausea
- Vomiting
- Tremors

**As for blood circulation problems caused by wearing tight clothes, the symptoms are:**

- Numbness
- Pain
- Change of skin color in affected area

## Symptoms of Raynaud's disease

- Coldness of affected body part
- Numbness

## Symptoms of lack of exercise

- Easy fatigability
- Lack of muscle tone
- Obesity or weight gain
- Unhealthy skin
- Claudication—pain in leg muscles when walking
- Slackened facial muscles—this can also be a symptom for MI
- Susceptibility to illnesses

You may experience the above-mentioned symptoms together with the symptoms of poor blood circulation or blocked circulation. Knowledge of all these symptoms will help you in determining the cause of your circulatory problem.

# Chapter 4: Treating Related Diseases

When prevention and natural cures are not sufficient in the management of your circulation problems, the last alternative is to make use of therapeutic drugs. Doctors will treat the root cause of your problem, while alleviating your symptoms. Treating the root cause will effectively solve your blood circulation problems. The following are methods used in treating these specific problems.

## Polycythemia vera

- **Blood extraction**—Because of the increased viscosity of blood, it has to be extracted to reduce your Red Blood Cells (RBCs). This reduction will render your blood less viscous.

- **Antihistamines**—These drugs are used in cases when itching becomes unbearable.

- **Anti-clotting or thinning drugs**—These will decrease the viscosity of your blood, allowing your blood to flow more freely through your circulatory system.

- **Hydroxyurea**—This is a drug class that reduces your RBCs. Remember that your

RBCs are abnormally high in numbers, so they must be reduced.

## Deep Venous thrombosis and Thrombophlebitis

- **Decompression clothing**—These are clothes that maintain a constant pressure on the affected areas so that formation of blood clots or thrombi is prevented.

- **Vein stripping**—This involves an invasive procedure where long varicose veins are "stripped" or removed.

- **Anti-clotting or thinning drugs**—These will eliminate thrombi or clot formation to promote blood flow. They are also called anticoagulants.

- **Thrombin inhibitors**—These will inhibit thrombin from being formed to prevent formation of clots that can clog the veins and arteries. When these don't work vena cava filters are used to filter out blood clots that can clog your circulatory system.

## Thrombocytopenia

- **Steroids**—These will reduce platelet destruction, so that the number of platelets in your blood will not lessen further. If it's a simple case of thrombocytopenia, your platelet count will go back to normal just by switching to a healthy diet and maintaining a healthy lifestyle.

- **Romiplostims**—These will help in the production of new platelets so that the count will return to its normal value.

- **Blood or platelet transfusions**—This is utilized when the condition is already severe, with values falling below 30,000/cumm. In this case, hemorrhage can occur, so transfusion must be done rapidly. This should be your last recourse though.

## Atherosclerosis and Arteriosclerosis

- **Statins**—The cause of this condition is elevated cholesterol levels therefore, you should take in medicines that lower the cholesterol in your body. However, dieting is the best course of action because statins have side effects that are detrimental to your health, too, such as muscle weakness. Examples are atorvastatin and fluvastatin.

- **Anti-clotting drugs**—This is to prevent clot formation in your blood vessels. Examples are aspirin, coumarin, cilostazol and pentoxifylline.

- **Angiotensin-Converting Enzyme (ACE) Inhibitors**—These help in reducing the progress of the condition. These are anti-hypertensive drugs that can also promote proper blood circulation.

- **Beta blockers and calcium channel blockers**—These are also anti-hypertensive drugs that help prevent the formation of clots, and aid in supporting smooth blood flow.

**Vertebrobasilar circulatory disorder**

- **Diet changes must be instituted**—Diet has a significant effect on the blood concentration of cholesterol that can cause vertebrobasilar circulatory disorder.

- **Hydrating fluids**—Water and hydrating fluids are given when dehydration occurs.

- **Statins**—If the root cause is atherosclerosis, the medicines used are the same as in the treatment for atherosclerosis.

- **Antihypertensive drugs**—Antihypertensive drugs such as those used for atherosclerosis (ACE inhibitors, beta blockers, and calcium channel blocking drugs) can be used.

- **Analgesics**—These are used for pain such as headaches, muscle pains and neck pains. Examples are paracetamol and aspirin.

- **Blood thinning drugs or anti-clotting drugs**—These are the drugs, including anticoagulants, also used in other blood circulatory conditions.

- **Antiemetics**—Drugs for vomiting and nausea are treated accordingly. Likewise with the other minor symptoms. Examples are plasil, tropisetron and dolasetron.

## Stress

- Stress should not require medication other than rest, relaxation and proper coping techniques. Medications should only be your last alternative.

- **Anti-anxiety drugs**—such as valium and trazepam are used in severe cases of stress.

### Raynaud's disease

- **Vasodilators**—These drugs enhance the widening of the blood vessels so that more blood can flow into your toes and fingers. As emphasized previously, all available natural treatment must be utilized first before using medicines. Examples are nitrostat, apresoline, natrecor and nitrogard

- **Calcium channel blockers**—These drugs will also widen the openings of the arteries to promote proper circulation. Examples are norvasc, procardia, isoptin, and cardene.

- **Beta blockers**—These drugs will dilate blood vessels, just like vasodilators and calcium channel blockers. Examples are metoprolol, neobloc, betaloc and nadolol.

- Warm up the affected areas and wear protective clothing.

### Peripheral arterial disease (PAD)

- **Anti-clotting drugs**—PAD can be treated by thinning or anti-clotting medication such as aspirin, cilostazol and pentoxifylline. These drugs are used to promote blood flow in the clogged blood vessels.

- **Surgery**—Angioplasty is a type of surgery that removes blocked arteries. However, you should only resort to surgery if natural treatment and drugs are not effective. Non-invasive or non-surgical procedures are still the best choices.

- The affected areas must be warmed and protected from cold temperatures.

### Herbal treatment

You can try herbal remedies such as ginkgo biloba, garlic, and ginger. These can be turned into concoctions that can be applied directly on the affected limb. You can also take them orally. They're not only good for circulatory problems but for general health, as well.

These are all the treatments used for the specific diseases related to blood circulation problems. As emphasized previously, use only medications when the natural methods are ineffective. Take note that even therapeutic drugs have side effects.

.

# Chapter 5: How to Improve Blood Circulation

Now that you know the major causes of problems in your blood circulation, you can now learn to prevent these from occurring. So, how do you improve your blood circulation? Here are methods you can implement.

## Step #1—Avoid bad cholesterol

One major cause of problems in your blood circulation is the accumulation of cholesterol or fats in your blood vessels. Cholesterol is a type of fat that should be present in your body in concentrations below 200 mg/dL only. To prevent the concentration of cholesterol from increasing, you have to avoid cholesterol-rich foods or fats. Elevated cholesterol concentrations can cause atherosclerosis, arteriosclerosis and hypertension. It also increases your risk of cardiac diseases such as MI and CVA, as mentioned in the previous chapter.

BUT—not all cholesterols are bad for you. There are bad cholesterols (Low Density Lipoproteins, LDL) and good cholesterols (High density Lipoproteins, HDL). The good cholesterols have crucial functions in your body that cannot be performed by other substances.

35

**Functions of good fat**

- **Serves as the basic nucleus of steroid hormones that include your sex hormones.** If you don't have cholesterol, you won't be able to develop your secondary sexual characteristics. You can imagine a world where there are no distinguishing physical traits between male and female. That's how important good cholesterol is.

- **Transports non-polar (water-hating substances) or water insoluble substances through the bloodstream in the form of Lipoproteins (LPP).** LPP acts as the boat that brings these non-polar substances to any part of the body where they are needed.

- **Acts as a bio membrane for major organs such as the brain and the lungs.** The bio membrane encloses these organs and protects them from easy injury and trauma. The phospholipids (good cholesterol) in your lungs make it possible for you to inhale and exhale. When the phospholipids are at an insufficient level, sudden death can occur just like with prematurely born babies who have incomplete lung development.

- **Acts as a heat insulator and helps the body maintain its temperature.** It's true that if you are fat, you should not feel cold easily because you have lots of insulation in your body. If you're fat and you still feel easily susceptible to cold temperatures, then you may have some pathological condition that simultaneously exists in your body.

- **Functions as a source of energy when carbohydrates are insufficient.** When it's used as a source of energy it can result to ketoacidosis in which ketone bodies are elevated in your body. This happens in diabetic patients who have insufficient insulin hormone to convert carbohydrates to energy.

We highlighted the primary functions of good cholesterol so you'll realize that fats have important functions in your body. Your body needs the good fats. That's why it's not enough that you learn about the good and bad fat, it's also vital that you know what food sources these types of fats come from so that you can stay healthy and fit.

### Sources of bad cholesterol

- Meat fats
- Egg yolks
- Other dairy products (Cheese and milk rich with fat)
- Vegetable shortening
- Liver

- Cream
- Refined sugar
- Trans or saturated fats
- Refined flour

Take note that food served in fast food chains are primary sources of bad fats. Your burgers and fries are rich sources of bad cholesterol.

## Sources of good cholesterol

- Dark green vegetables such as lettuce, spinach, broccoli, collard greens and mustard greens
- Olive oil
- Fruits such as watermelon, banana, avocado, guava, lemon and papaya
- Fish oil (cod liver oil)
- Plant oils such as sunflower oil, and flaxseed oil
- Oats
- Whole grains
- Legumes

Eat more of the food that provides good cholesterol, if you want to improve your blood circulation—eat more fruits and vegetables.

Now that you know these facts, you have to put this valuable information into use by conscientiously choosing your meals.

## Step #2—Exercise daily

You may have heard a million times that exercise is good for your health. It's a fact that you cannot run away from because exercising daily is an essential part of the daily regimen for those who want to stay healthy and promote proper circulation in their bodies.

Your exercise need not be strenuous or high-grade. What's important is that you do it within the recommended time, which is from 30 minutes to 1 hour, and you do it consistently. You can choose a light exercise regimen that you can easily commit to do daily. The exercise must be able to let you sweat and increase your respiration and heartbeat.

With the increase of your respiration and heartbeat, the blood circulation in your body increases too, making it possible for the increased flow of blood to "flush" accumulated fats or substances from your blood vessels. This will promote the smooth flow of your blood through all your cells, tissues and organs. Exercise has been proven to relieve stress as well.

**Suggestions for daily exercises:**

- Walking
- Swimming
- Cycling
- Aerobics
- Jogging
- Dancing

If you don't have time to set aside specifically for daily exercise, incorporate activities in your daily routine. Maybe you can bike to work, jog or walk when doing errands, etc. If you can't afford a full hour work out in one go, you can go walking on a staggered basis by taking 15-minute walks every break time until you complete one hour.

You may not realize it, but the exercises that you do daily are your life-savers!

**Step #3—Dress appropriately**

Above dressing fashionably, your comfort and health should still be your priority when choosing your clothing. Select clothes that don't restrict the flow of blood to any part of your body. When blood vessels are obstructed, this can result to syncope (fainting) and serious effects that can result to death. Avoid tight-fitting pants, leggings, and jewelries that clamp tightly on your arms or legs. Who needs fashion that will place your health in danger?

In cold regions where Raynaud's disease can be exacerbated, you must wear gloves or socks to protect your extremities from the cold. Compression clothing can also help in cases of thrombophlebitis and venous thrombosis.

## Step #4—Avoid stressful situations

Stress can increase your risk of circulatory problems. This is due to the fact that stress can result in hormone responses that impede blood circulation. One example is that when you're stressed out, you may feel a lump in your throat or butterflies in your stomach. These are genuine symptoms that can constrict your blood vessels and cause problems. The hormones produced are explained in chapter 2.

But since a small amount of stress is a normal part of daily activities, you can also learn how to cope with it by learning some relaxation techniques. A simple way to do this every day is to perform breathing exercises. Below is a simple exercise you can do quickly.

## Simple breathing exercise

- Stand or sit with your back straight.

- Close your eyes and place your arms akimbo.

- Breathe in deeply through your nose, taking note of how your rib cage lifts up and how your chest expands. Feel the air entering your nose and into your lungs.

- Hold your breath for 7 seconds.

- Breathe out forcibly through your mouth. Notice how your rib cage lowers and your chest relaxes. Feel the air leaving your body.

- Mentally psyche yourself to relax.

- Do this several times until you feel your muscles relax and your breathing become stable.

- You can do this anytime and anywhere, whenever you feel stressed out. Doing it twice a day is typically enough.

You can learn more complex relaxation techniques such as Yoga, Transcendental Meditation or Mindful Meditation. But even this simple breathing exercise is incredibly helpful and sufficiently effective.

## Step #5—Avoid drugs that thins blood

Heparin, Coumadin and aspirin are blood thinners. They reduce the viscosity of blood, usually to prevent formation of clots. However, too much of it can do the opposite—blood turns less viscous which results in wounds no longer clotting, thus putting you at risk of bleeding to death, if not treated immediately. To avoid circulation problems in this case, you have to get the consent of your doctor before taking these drugs.

## Step #6—Refrain from vices

Refrain from drinking alcohol, smoking cigarettes, and doing drugs. These are all substances of abuse that are detrimental to your health. Anything unhealthy can cause circulatory problems. The caffeine in coffee can also be addictive, so don't indulge in coffee during breaks. You can enjoy non-caffeinated coffee instead.

## Step #7—Visit your doctor annually

Getting a regular check-up annually—even if you don't feel there's anything wrong—is a superb way to maintain your health. Of course, if you notice the symptoms appearing, you have to consult your doctor ASAP. Don't wait for things to get out of hand before springing to action. It's better to be safe than sorry.

These are simple steps that you can implement if you want to prevent problems with your blood circulation. Observe these preventive measures and you'll improve your natural inclination for avoiding health problems.

# Chapter 6: Valuable Tips for a Healthier Body

The significance of healthy blood circulation can never be discounted. In fact, it's your existing lifeline. Without it, you won't be able to live or function normally. Therefore, knowing all there is to know about this precious lifeline, puts you at an advantage. Here are additional pointers to ensure that you maintain a healthy circulatory system.

1. **A body massage has good effects on blood circulation**. You can pamper yourself once in a while by undergoing a relaxing body massage. For sure, massage also helps relieve your stress.

2. **Excess intake of sugar (glucose from carbohydrates), particularly under diabetic conditions can aggravate blood circulation problems.** The excess sugar in your body can slow down the flow of blood because of increased viscosity.

3. **The cause and effect can be a two-way traffic.** The cause of blood circulation problems can sometimes become the effect.

An example is your atherosclerosis; it can be the cause and it can also become the effect.

4. **When taking a bath, use lukewarm water.** It should be moderately warm, neither too hot nor too cold. Extreme temperatures can worsen your condition. But, if your extremities get cold, you can use hot water bags to warm them.

5. **Avoid remaining in one position for long periods of time.** Shift your body position every now and then. In the evenings, elevate your legs to rest them.

6. **Remember to keep hydrated.** Drink lots of water because it is a universal solvent that can help flush out those toxic substances. This will also allow your blood cells to function properly.

7. **A combination of prevention and treatment techniques is the best.** You have to combine compatible methods to resolve your circulatory problems effectively.

8.  **Pregnant mothers have an increased risk of poor circulation in the legs.** This is due to arteries being blocked by the pregnancy.

9.  **Obesity and overweight individuals have a greater propensity towards circulatory problems**. This is because excess fat can block veins and arteries.

10. **Acupuncture, reflexology and hydrotherapy can be used to treat blood circulation problems.** More and more studies point to the effectiveness of these alternative methods.

# Conclusion

The majority of blood circulation problems can be prevented by living a healthy life. Being aware of this can help you overcome circulation problems and manage existing ones.

In summary, the key to the prevention of blood circulation problems is exercise, correct diet, enough sleep, and sufficient water intake. Avoiding drugs of abuse that can harm the body is also a given, if you want to stay healthy.

Implementing all the techniques from this book will definitely prevent blood circulation problems. Don't wait for disease to strike. Share the information with your family, follow these techniques and live a life free from circulatory problems.

Finally, I'd like to thank you for purchasing this book! If you found it helpful, I'd greatly appreciate it if you'd take a moment to leave a review on Amazon. Thank you!

Printed in Great Britain
by Amazon

33797928R00036